Just Decide!

Just Decide!

A Guide to Your Body, Mind & Spirit Agreements

CARRIE BROOKS

IGUANA

Disclaimer: This is a work inspired by real-life events. In certain cases incidents, names and timelines have been changed for dramatic purposes. Certain names may be composites or entirely fictitious. Identifying characteristics and details have been changed as well.

This book is designed to provide entertainment to readers. It is shared and sold with the understanding that the author is not engaged to render any type of psychological, medical, legal, or any other kind of personal or professional advice. No warranties or guarantees are expressed or implied by the author's choice to include any of the content in this volume. The reader should always consult his or her medical, health, or other professional and accredited health provider before adopting any of the suggestions in this book or drawing any ideas, inferences, or practices from this book. The author shall not be liable for any physical, psychological, emotional, financial, or commercial damages, including, but not limited to, special, incidental, consequential, or other damages. The reader is responsible for their own choices, actions, and results.

Publisher: Meghan Behse
Editor: Paula Chiarcos
Front cover design: Ruth Dwight, designplayground.ca

ISBN 978-1-77180-488-2 (paperback)
ISBN 978-1-77180-489-9 (epub)

This is an original print edition of *Just Decide! A Guide to Your Body, Mind & Spirit Agreements*.

*To my family, for being my main source of
inspiration and experience as well as my
greatest sense of love, joy, and fulfillment.
Much love.*

CONTENTS

Preface

I didn't love high school, aside from time with friends. I've never been good at being told what to do, and the silly teenage hierarchy really pissed me off. The friendships and shared experiences though, most importantly with Mike, my husband of almost twenty-five years, are my most cherished high school memories.

I went into Early Childhood Education and did great because it was my choice and my interest. I worked in that field for two years and left after a discussion with Mike because we knew we wanted children, but I couldn't imagine working with and raising children simultaneously ... I have a great deal of respect for teachers and really don't know how they do it!

About a year later, Mike and I were married. Within four years we had our daughter, Sierra, and our son, Jake, just after moving into our first house. I couldn't believe how complete I felt having accomplished my largest aspirations to date. That was the summary, at the time, of my life's ambitions. Now what? I always wanted to work with people so I took a variety of jobs until I realized what I wanted to do.

At the same time, the change in my physical appearance and feelings of fatigue after my kids were born felt foreign and uncomfortable. My weight had never been so high, and I didn't like it one bit. After deciding to make changes to my diet by placing an emphasis on whole and colourful foods, I reviewed and established appropriate portion control. I used images and articles from fitness magazines for motivation and direction; then when I achieved the body image that I had worked so hard for, I decided to share my energy and accomplishments with others.

I completed my Certified Personal Trainer theoretical and practical course in the fall of 2001, roughly eighteen months after the birth of my second child. In February 2002, I began training clients at a local gym in Cambridge, Ontario ... some are still with me. Since then I've competed in two fitness competitions and took countless additional courses to further my knowledge of wellness. Finally, I have to mention that I wrote this book during the Covid-19 pandemic, and that experience was part of what inspired me. I felt out of sorts at the beginning. For the first time, I was laid off and it simply wasn't a comfortable feeling. But I always wanted to lead, inspire, and motivate others to feel great, so increasing my reach during this difficult time felt like an awesome idea!

I hope this book will guide and assist you in developing new *agreements* through action and repetition (more on *agreements* later). The beginning of this process is the book title: First you must *Just Decide!* It's completely up to you! So why not feel better?

Introduction

Like many of you, my exercise choices and activity level have evolved over the years. Early on, I adopted a trial-and-error approach, and I favour health and wellness *guidelines* over strict adherence to *rules*. In my experience there isn't a one-size-fits-all program, and I truly believe there's a way to make wellness and exercise enjoyable for everybody who wants it. I mean, after all, it's *your* body! So of course you ought to care for it in *your* way, right?

Just think about it … As children, our caregivers were responsible for our protection and wellness. Some *agreements* were made *for* us at that formative time in our lives. By agreements, I mean conscious and subconscious decisions that we've made or "agreed" to. For example, growing up in my house, the expectation was to "finish all the food on your plate because there are children who are hungry." As adults, aside from the professional advice and healthcare we seek, it's our responsibility to make the best decisions and take the right action so that we thrive.

The intention of this book is to show you how to improve your body, mind, and spirit so that *you* can make new agreements for yourself.

I'll help you recognize the action your *body* provides, the decision that your *mind* provides, and the feelings that your *spirit* provides to develop your new agreements. But it begins with you. You are the only one with control over what you think, do, and feel. Although this is difficult for some to believe, really consider this statement. Others can inspire our thoughts, tell us what to do, and evoke feelings in us, but we alone have *control over what we think, do, and feel.* It's simple but not easy.

I've given you some space in most sections so you can write your thoughts. In order to get the most out of my book, keep the following in mind when you're journaling:

1. Search your mind and don't hold back.
2. Incorporate emotion or "the feels" to increase the energy of the written word.

So, let's get motivated! I'm going to help you figure out what you want and the steps to take to get there so you can be the best version of you. It's your body. Own it.

I do *me,* and you do *you.*

Me: *Motivate*; *Empower.*

You: *Yes* (agreement); *Outsource* specialized knowledge; *Understand.*

Agreed?

PART I
Body

CHAPTER 1
Your body, your vessel

Let's dive right in! There's no mistaking the importance of water for our survival and optimal wellness. In fact, your *vessel* is completely dependent on water. You're made of roughly 60–70% water, and while your body can typically survive without food for about three weeks, the absence of water after about three days can lead to organ failure, fainting, strokes, and death. While this result is extreme, adequate daily intake of water is very important as it supports and nourishes many of your body's systems and functions.

Saliva is made up predominantly of water and it's an essential component of digestion. Regular fluid intake assists your body in the production of saliva, but production can decrease through the ageing process, medications, or therapies (Silver 2020). So we need to drink even more water as we age. Drinking water may also activate your metabolism thereby increasing your energy. Water also helps with nutrient absorption by dissolving vitamins, minerals, and other nutrients from your food then delivering them to the rest of your body. By carrying helpful nutrients and oxygen to our entire body, water improves our circulation and therefore has a positive impact on our overall health. It even helps protect your tissues, spinal cord, and joints by lubricating them. This can lessen discomfort during physical activity and aid in mobility. Since we're built to move, why not make it feel better?

Adequate hydration is also imperative to your body's temperature control. During physical activity, stress, and hot weather, your body loses water through sweat in order to keep cool. So you have to drink more water to maintain that temperature regulation and avoid dehydration (Silver 2020). This has the added benefit of improving physical performance. By replacing fluids lost through sweat during exercise, you'll have more strength, power, and endurance.

Did you know that studies have linked body fat and weight loss with the amount of water you drink (Bjarnadottir 2020)? Water fills your stomach and helps prevent overeating. It also aids in the release of waste through proper digestion, and it helps your kidneys work more efficiently. In other words, you need enough water in your system to excrete waste and avoid constipation. Shit happens right? No need for it to be painful.

Adequate water intake also helps improve mood and cognitive function. In fact, dehydration can result in fatigue, confusion, anxiety, and an inability to focus. And how about this for a bonus: Water helps keep your skin hydrated and bright. Consider it an ingestible (and cheap!) moisturizer that helps to reduce the effects of ageing (Silver 2020).

So, how much should we drink each day? The suggested amount of water required daily is ½ to 1 ounce per pound of bodyweight. This is quite a variance since a person weighing 150 pounds should drink 75 to 150 ounces … Perhaps a better rule of thumb would be to just pay attention to your body. Feeling thirsty and having dark-yellow urine are symptoms of dehydration, so if you experience either of these, you should have a drink of water. And if you find these things are happening a lot, that means you should up your intake even more.

There are more types of drinking water than many imagine (Still 2009):

- Tap water is safe to drink in many countries; check out your local water regulatory authority.
- Mineral water comes from a spring and provides, you guessed it, minerals!
- Spring or glacier waters also contain minerals, though some are untested.
- Sparkling plain water offers fizz without added sugars — unless flavoured.
- Distilled water is boiled, steam-collected, and condensed back to liquid — a clean option where water might be contaminated.

- Purified water is tap or groundwater that is processed to remove contaminants.
- Flavoured water has added flavourings and sweeteners.
- Well water from dug or drilled wells should be tested and/or treated.

This list is not necessarily complete, but as you can see, there are lots of choices! So try a few out. See what you like. Add your own flavour with fresh fruit or herbs, like citrus or mint. Commit to having water by you and sip throughout the day. So ... how much water do you intend to drink daily?

_____

_____

_____

Following through on this decision with consistent action will make it a habit. You've just got to decide to do it.

Cheers!

Agreed?

CHAPTER 2
Ya gotta eat!

Thank goodness, right? I'm a big fan of flavourful food and enjoying my meals. I've been known to do a little food dance and/or hum while eating. This is why I offer suggestions and guidelines *instead of* strict adherence to a set diet or meal plan. Before going forward I'd like to illustrate my preferred definition of that four-letter word.

Diet: food regularly consumed by a person; habitual nourishment.

It doesn't need to be construed in a negative way!

I've followed many restrictive plans and found that while there may be a period of success, the strict limitations feel too rigid to maintain in the long term. The second challenge of absolute restrictions is losing flexibility when travelling or dining out. Of course this is less of a concern during the Covid-19 pandemic, but that's bound to change.

Ultimately, the decision is yours! For those who enjoy the structure and direction of diet and meal plans, they can be easily found. Likely in the very section that you found this book. There are also many food services that will deliver wholesome and pre-packaged meals or whole foods to your door. We find some guidelines or rules helpful because structure aids in meal-planning and offers comfort. The lure of success, whatever that means to you, is what grabs our attention and eager participation (for a time) with all diets. And the primary reason most people bail on their diet is that they become frustrated when they don't see quick results. Consider the post you've likely seen on social media or any media for that matter: "I've been on this diet for two whole days and my pants aren't falling off." Please, please, please have some patience! Your body didn't develop overnight and it certainly won't change that quickly either. As I'm not suggesting adherence to any specific diet but rather offering information, I'll simply list as many diets as I can with minimal explanation. In no particular order...

- Whole foods: unprocessed or minimally processed foods.
- Paleo: hunter-gatherer style without processed foods.
- Raw food: whole uncooked foods or heated to 48°C max.
- Carnivore: 100% food from animals.

- Vegan: non-animal foods.
- Lacto-vegetarian: vegetarian plus milk products.
- Ovo-vegetarian: vegetarian plus eggs.
- Lacto-ovo-vegetarian: vegetarian plus milk products and eggs.
- Pescatarian: vegetarian plus fish and seafood.
- Pollotarian: vegetarian plus chicken and eggs.
- Flexitarian: whole foods with flexibility to include animal products.
- Mediterranean: whole foods, grains, moderate dairy, limited red meat.
- Low carb: limited starchy carbs and refined carbohydrates.
- The 100 Mile: locally sourced foods.

Which, if any, of these is closest to your current diet? Journal your meals in the space below, including approximate serving sizes and foods for the last week. If you can't remember, then journal your recent norms.

_____

_____

_____

_____

_____

_____

_____

_____

_____

_____

_____

_____

_____

_____

_____

_____

_____

_____

_____

_____

_____

_____

_____

_____

_____

_____

_____

_____

_____

_____

_____

_____

_____

_____

I've found that people have some favourite foods and eating practices. That being said, you're likely reading this because you want to change your body in some way. Making changes to your body (or anything for that matter) requires a change in your action and habits. As stated earlier, it's repetitive action that becomes a habit. So how can we better prepare ourselves for that action? Well, don't bite off more than you can chew ... so to speak.

So ... avid steak lover, feel like trying vegetarianism? I'd say that's unlikely. And I'd probably get the same answer from a vegetarian being offered a steak.

So how do you change your diet but keep it *your* diet? My consistent suggestion (simply because it allows for individual interpretation) is **a whole food diet that is rich in colour and variety**. Also, because I'm the author and have carte blanche, *please stop, stop, stop villainizing food groups!* Badmouthing "carbs" when you mean starchy or processed and refined carbohydrates is incorrect. Broccoli is a carb, people! Ok, end rant.

Another important factor is *when* you eat your meals. There are a few reasons for this. I don't want to drive you crazy with textbook or "sciencey" language, so I'll offer simple and brief explanations for some of our body's functions:

The mechanical portion of the digestive system begins when you eat, or specifically, when you put food in your mouth. Your saliva has enzymes that assist in the breaking down of food while you chew. Remember the saying "Chew your food well." I can't imagine how those champion speed eaters perform such tasks without indigestion. This mechanical process continues through your esophagus, stomach, small intestine, and large intestine, and ends with waste excretion.

Metabolism is the chemical reaction in your body's cells that changes food to energy, which is used to keep the systems of your body functioning and for the actions you perform. The speed of metabolism (metabolic rate) indicates your calorie expenditure (calories burned). Some factors that affect metabolism are ageing, muscle mass, body size, temperature regulation, and physical activity. Another consideration is the defence mechanism of *starvation mode* wherein your metabolism slows in response to prolonged caloric deficit — measured in days, not hours.

And as if you haven't heard enough about hormones throughout your life, did you know that hormones also play many roles during chemical digestion and following it? There are lots of books and websites that explain this process well. I checked out rejoovwellness.com and also learned a lot from the book, *The Obesity Code*, by Dr. Jason Fung. Basically, some responsibilities of your gut hormones are to regulate appetite, gut mobility, and energy metabolism. A key player in this metabolism is insulin, which is released from the pancreas after eating to help convert blood sugar into energy for immediate use. Anything not immediately used is stored in your muscles and liver as glycogen. When those stores are full, glucose is converted into fatty acids and stored in adipose tissue — fat (Mangano 2011). So … insulin converts food to energy for immediate use, then your body stores glycogen, then it stores fat.

Under normal conditions, low insulin levels encourage glycogen and fat burning, aka *fat loss*. This is what the majority of you want. Times of insulin absence allow you to be sensitive to it and allow it to do its job. It's kinda like you need some insulin *absence* to be *fond* of it. But persistently high insulin levels over a prolonged period can cause an increase in insulin resistance, which makes it harder for your body to turn blood sugar into usable energy and remove it from the bloodstream. This can occur if you eat too often (grazing) or not often enough (starvation mode). So what should you do? First, let's figure out how often you eat.

Like many of you, I've tried the two most popular options:

1. Smaller and more frequent meals and snacks spaced 2 to 3 hours apart, totalling five or six per day. At one time, it was believed that this *grazing* type of meal plan would prevent metabolism from slowing down. However, studies have shown mixed results and it's unclear if this is the case. In fact, some studies suggest that consistent *grazing* can elicit a more constant presence of insulin (Virgin 2013).

2.   Three meals per day spaced roughly 4 hours apart (traditional breakfast, lunch, and dinner). Known as *intermittent fasting*, the premise here is that spacing meals apart to allow for more digestion time, as well as an extended fasting period between dinner one day and breakfast the next, allows for low insulin levels, which encourages your body to burn glycogen and fat.

Perhaps you remember my aforementioned love of food? This is not accompanied, sadly, by a love of cooking. So I favour *intermittent fasting*.

Which one of these is closest to your current meal schedule? Consider the timing of your meals for the past week. Return to your food journal and, if you haven't already done so, add the times of day when you ate. Keeping in mind that a change to your body requires a change to your habits and actions, what do you notice? Do any changes appear necessary? If so, record them below. If you prefer guidance, then outsource to a health professional.

_____

_____

_____

_____

_____

_____

_____

Did you write a few things? Maybe many things? Are you eating out of habit or because you're hungry or bored? Oftentimes, hunger isn't the driving force for eating. Consider how your eating habits differ when you go to à la carte restaurants versus buffet-style restaurants. What about social interactions where food is readily available — are you eating because you're hungry or because it's there, it's yummy, or you just feel it's impolite to say no thanks. Knowing *why* you eat is just as important as what you eat. Food is enjoyable fuel for our bodies. I want you to enjoy it while choosing the guidelines that serve you best. So cut out the boredom, comfort, and polite eating. Does that lead you to three or four meals spaced evenly throughout your day? Give that a go then and see how it feels and works for ya!

Remember, it's best not to bite off more than you can chew. So choose one or two changes at a time and practise as best you can until they become a habit. Did you get that? 1) *Actively practise* and 2) *as best you can.* In order to see results, guidelines must be *actively practised* for a period of time that will vary from person to person. For most, if an activity is kept up for about 21 days it starts to become a habit. But let's be realistic. Following guidelines with absolute precision and perfection is not the life that I want to live or the one I would suggest for you. Choosing to follow them *as best you can* means exactly that. Ideally, while you're seeking changes to your body, follow the 80/20 rule. If you're eating 3 meals per day (so 21 meals per week) the rule allows for 4 meals per week that don't follow your guidelines. 21 meals x 20% = 4. If you're eating more meals per week, simply change the math. These changes to your diet will be the base of your long-term meal plan. The longer you adhere to them, so long as they serve you well, the easier they will become.

Agreed?

CHAPTER 3

Creating habits: Doing something over and over and over ... until it sticks

Pretty simple statement here: *repetitious action creates habit.* The fact that you're reading this indicates you have an interest in feeling better and developing new habits. You decided that you want to read this book and you're currently following through with action. Every habit you have was cemented by repetitive action. Did anyone tell you to push back the bedding before rising from bed this morning? What about washing your hands after your morning flush? Of course these are simple and mindless for most of us (I hope), but after being taught these habits we agreed to them. New agreements become natural to us through repetitive action.

I've talked about the importance of water and wholesome nutrition at the appropriate meal intervals to serve you. Now that you've decided on three primary changes, you'll need to ... can you guess? Take action!!

I'm suggesting three at a time to avoid the feeling of

being overwhelmed by change. And remember to use the "21-day, as best you can" strategy from the previous chapter. So follow them daily until they become natural to you or until *no conscious thought is required*. When you feel like these are habits, it's time to add other changes and/or edit things that aren't serving you well. For example, if you've chosen to delay breakfast in efforts to follow a 16-hour fast and 8-hour eating window of *intermittent fasting* but you're getting headaches, then change the timing. Perhaps a 14-hour fast and a 10-hour eating window is the right way to ease in. What are your three primary agreements?

_____

_____

_____

_____

_____

_____

_____

_____

_____

_____

_____

_____

_____

_____

_____

_____

_____

_____

_____

_____

_____

_____

_____

_____

It's important to keep in mind that developing new behaviors and habits will take some time. Simply do your best. If you falter, then begin again. All or nothing is a piss-poor approach because inconveniences and surprises happen. Make consistent efforts to commit or recommit to your agreements daily until they're a natural habit ... like the aforementioned handwashing! When a habit or *agreement* becomes set then begin work on another.

In the mind section of this book, we'll get deeper into how these habits are created — because the mind is where habits begin, through brainstorming, decision-making, repetitive affirmations, and action. Affirmations are designed to inspire action and the days and weeks that follow are the necessary work that turn these decisions into new habits or *agreements*. This chapter is short and sweet because action is about doing!

Agreed?

CHAPTER 4
Fun with fitness

Yup, that's what I said. How often have you done things you didn't enjoy because they were *good for you*? To help make the actions doable, why not find a way to enjoy them? If, for example, exercise is new to you I'd highly suggest trying things that sound fun. Maybe you've heard friends, family, or colleagues speaking of activities they've enjoyed and you'd like to give them a try. Great! If you enjoy working as a team or in a group then that's a good way to start. If solitude feels better to you, then so be it!

Of course, through habit and the great feelings that accompany wellness, you'll very likely come to enjoy some aspect of your exercise routine. Maybe you'll appreciate the feeling of strength when you can lift or move something that was previously too difficult, or the camaraderie that you feel when working out with a partner or a group, or the feeling of stability when you put on a shoe while standing on one leg. I mean the list is endless.

In the twenty years that I've been motivating and educating clients, I've heard so many reasons why they decided they wanted to gain an improved level of wellness in the physical realm:

I want to feel stronger.
I want to decrease my waistline.
I want the energy to play with my kids or grandkids.
I want my arms to jiggle less when I wave.
I want to recover from an injury.
I want my body to feel more firm.
I want to look better.

I could continue this list for many pages, and maybe I haven't touched on *your* want, but it's my intent to help you define it and develop an action plan. We'll get into that more in Part II when we talk about your mind. For now, use the space provided to jot down or doodle some of your wants.

_____

_____

_____

_____

_____

_____

_____

_____

_____

_____

_____

_____

_____

_____

_____

_____

_____

_____

_____

_____

_____

Make no mistake, I'm not here to tell you what to do. I'm here to motivate and empower. What's important from **YOU** is **Y**es (agreement); **O**utsource specialized knowledge; **U**nderstand the information you find. I'll repeat strategies throughout this book to open your mind to the endless possibilities you have.

What I want to introduce you to, or maybe enlighten you more about, are the great many types and styles of exercise options. In no particular order, here we go!

INDEPENDENT STRENGTH & FLOW EXERCISES

No surprise that this style is first on my list since these are some of my favourites and how I've predominantly been training myself and clients for twenty years. Included in these exercises are bodyweight training, strength training with a variety of free weights or equipment, boot-camp style or obstacle course workouts (think G.I. Jane), High Intensity Interval Training (HIIT), yoga, and Pilates. The exercises included in these styles are damn near limitless, so if something here piques your interest and you're not familiar with it then talk to your local trainer/instructor or look it up on the internet.

TRAIL OR TRACK FUN

Lace up and go! Like many of you, in the past year I've done more walking than ever before. It's kinda like an active outdoor fashion show 'cause all you need is the right outfit (weather appropriate) and footwear. Change up the scenery from your neighbourhood to a local track or trail. Want a greater challenge? Perhaps empower the Tigger in you with some hurdles. When you're ready for an extra challenge, you can change your pace: walk — jog — run — sprint. And keep striving for that ideal posture — just imagine a string holding you erect like that well-adjusted marionette in the Robaxacet commercial.

FIELD ATHLETICS

These remind me of school days. On a field you can throw: javelin, discus, shot put, or hammer. And you can leap: long jump, triple jump, high jump, or pole vault. Alternatively, if you'd like to get in touch with your inner warrior you can SHOOT … an arrow. Archery is a fun activity that I did with Mike after the birth of our daughter as a bring-the-baby-along date 'cause she would sit happily (and safely) strapped in her chair watching us. We used a recurve bow and a compound bow, and there are more to choose from. Beyond these activities, countless sports can be played on a field with a few or many people. Consider football, soccer, lacrosse, field hockey, baseball, or softball, to name a few.

FUN ON WHEELS

Remember the saying "It's like riding a bike…" Most of us have been riding bikes since we were little, but maybe one of these styles is new to you: upright or recumbent stationary, mountain, hybrid/comfort, road, triathlon/time-trial, BMX/trick, commuting, cyclocross, track/fixed gear, tandem, adult trike, folding, or beach cruiser. You can also stand on wheels with roller or inline skates, skateboards, longboards, or penny boards. I have super fond memories of Dad taking my brother and me to Skate Country so we could whip around the roller rink to cool tunes and lights!

BODY WEIGHT EXERCISES

Many classically known exercises using body weight are great challenges. Because there's no equipment necessary, it's a versatile option that can be employed almost anywhere to give you a full-body workout. Ideas include but are not limited to the following:

- Squats
- Planks
- Bench dips
- Burpees
- Lunges
- Lateral leg raises
- Glute bridges
- Mountain climbers
- Skater hops
- Hip extensions
- Standing oblique crunches
- Jumping jacks
- Push-ups

RACQUET SPORTS

Tennis was another go-to for me growing up after my parents joined a local tennis club and set me up with some lessons — thanks Mom and Dad! Not limited to tennis however, you could try squash, racquetball, table tennis, or Ping-Pong — even if you don't become famous like Forrest Gump did in the 2013 movie of the same name. For those who don't recognize the reference, Ping-Pong existed way before beer pong!

GOLF (NOT JUST FOR GRANDPARENTS ANYMORE)

When I was growing up, golf was thought of as a grandparent activity — perhaps because my grandparents played, but it was also the general consensus. That is certainly not the case anymore! You can hit the links on a public or private course with equipment rented, borrowed, or bought. Eighteen holes or perhaps just nine to start? Practise your swing at outdoor or indoor driving ranges or lighten up a little with some mini-golf. I've found both are fun with friends!

WATER ACTIVITIES

Find some water and jump in! Swimming in open water provides beautiful scenery and the added challenge of flowing water, which might pique your interest. If not, then many communities have indoor and outdoor pools for public use. Don't want to submerge? While there's no actual guarantee of that, you could strap on a life vest and try some on-water sports: canoeing, kayaking, surfing, or paddleboarding. Learning to steer and balance has created some comical memories for me. Most recently, falling into the lake (my justification for the use of life vests) while learning to use a paddleboard last summer — I'll definitely do it again!

ADVENTURE SPORTS

Are you a thrill seeker? (Me, not so much.) While all sports require varying levels of skill, adventure sports tend to include an element of danger. Examples include rock or mountain climbing, hang gliding, parasailing, skydiving or parachuting, zip-lining, bungee jumping, whitewater rafting, scuba diving, horse riding, and Zorbing. I've tried two of these and can honestly say that while they were exciting, they offered more stimulation than I require. And remember, adventure sports can be risky, so practise caution while you're having fun!

COMBAT SPORTS

Boxing, karate, tae kwon do, and jiu-jitsu are examples of combat sports. Far beyond self-defence, they offer self-mastery, skill, and honour. By no means am I seeking to minimize this point but ... remember Mr. Miyagi from *The Karate Kid* films? He sought not only to teach defence and striking skills but also respect, balance, breathing, and understanding over knowledge. Quality life skills and a workout ... sign me up!

WINTER SPORTS

Downhill skiing, snowboarding, and luge can also be classified as adventure sports, but since they occur in winter, I've decided to include them here. Gravity and a slick or snow-covered surface can really amp up your speed. (Guess how many I've tried?) My brother tried to teach me to snowboard at a modest local hill and I learned that gravity wins over balance more often than I enjoy — for the activity to continue regularly that is. The time with him was the best part of that experience! For less of a speedy gravitational challenge, you could try cross-country skiing or snowshoeing, remembering that neither are a "walk in the park!"

Albeit extensive, this list is far from complete and maybe you've got other activities that you'd like to try.

That's great and I highly encourage you to take immediate and consistent action to cement healthy new habits. Go ahead and record in the space below the activities that piqued your interest.

_____

_____

_____

_____

_____

_____

_____

_____

_____

_____

_____

_____

_____

_____

_____

_____

_____

Time to move it! What will you try first? Don't overthink it, go with your gut. The first part of this exercise process is absolutely up to you, *Just Decide!*
Agreed?

CHAPTER 5

Almighty sleep

Where to begin about this powerful need we have ... oh, I know, how about bright-eyed and bushy-tailed in the morning! That fabulous feeling we get when we've had a great night's sleep that helps us to start the day with a feeling of invincibility.

But how much sleep is enough? Of course it varies person to person and day to day, and while illness and injury can affect our sleep needs, most healthy adults require between 7 and 9 hours every night. You likely know your requirements based on how you feel, think, and perform following varying amounts of sleep. And because most of us aren't living in an ideally scheduled way, we simply need to strive for our *best rest scenario*.

So, how do we get there? Developing a consistent sleep routine is a great idea! Here are a few ideas to get you started:

- Gentle evening activity — walking, yoga, meditation, etc.

- Absence of snacking after dinner — your body can't digest and properly rest simultaneously.
- Absence of caffeine later in the day.
- Conflict resolution — settling all that you can and dismissing from mind that which you cannot.
- Calmness leading up to bedtime — whatever this means to you.
- Avoidance of blue light in the evening.
- A consistent bedtime routine — personal hygiene habits.
- Regular or consistent sleeping hours — bedtime and wake time.
- Sleep comfort — bedding, absence of lighting, temperature.
- Waking with gratitude — positive thoughts.
- Refreshing morning routine — meditation, stretches, a shower.

Does any of this sound familiar to you? Consider your current sleep routine (as recent as last night) and record it below.

_____

_____

_____

_____

_____

_____

_____

_____

_____

_____

_____

_____

_____

_____

What, if anything, would you like to change to establish your *best rest scenario*? Scratch out habits that you don't believe are helpful to you then record your new plan here.

_____

_____

_____

_____

_____

_____

_____

_____

_____

_____

_____

_____

_____

Growth, development, and repair occurs during sleep with the aid of human growth hormone (HGH). Your body naturally produces HGH and the majority is released in pulses as you sleep. Inadequate or poor sleep can reduce the amount of HGH your body produces. The amount also decreases gradually as we age, but there are some habits we can adopt to help slow the decrease.

First, you can adjust your eating habits so that your insulin levels are lower at night. Why? Well remember in Chapter 2, we talked about insulin and how it's released as a result of eating (and note that foods having the greatest or highest insulin response are refined carbs and/or sugars). This means that if you don't snack between dinner and bedtime (especially sugary snacks) you'll be more likely to sleep without the presence of insulin, and this is a good thing because studies have shown insulin decreases the production and release of HGH (Mawer 2019).

no snacking = lower insulin = higher levels of HGH at night = better sleep

The second way you can keep your HGH levels higher is through exercise, which can create a spike in HGH. All exercise is beneficial, though High Intensity Interval Training (HIIT), which involves bursts of activity blended with rest periods using a variety of exercises and timing patterns, creates the greatest response in HGH levels. A standard routine is 20 seconds of exercise followed by 10 seconds of rest — repeated eight times for a total of 4 minutes. Think, squats — rest — push-ups — rest. If HIIT isn't something you're ready for, no problem, because the list of choices in chapter 4 is vast, and through trial and error you're sure to find some favourites!

At one point or another, sleep eludes all of us. But it's so important, it's worth aiming for that 7 to 9 hours per night. Sleep allows relaxation and restoration in between our daily activities, and our *best rest scenario* gives us the greatest potential to get adequate amounts of deep sleep. Review and practise your *best rest scenario* daily to ensure optimal levels of HGH ... it's referred to as beauty sleep for a reason, ya know!

Agreed?

PART II
Mind

CHAPTER 6
Strengthen your mind too!

In Part I we talked about how to strengthen your body — but that's not where strength is born. It occurs first in your mind. Why is it important to build strength in our minds, you ask? Because building our resilience or mental toughness better enables us to overcome obstacles and recover from difficulties. It's about problem-solving, ya know? Problem-solving is not only a tool for the continued strengthening of your mind but also supports your wellness plan. When following a wellness plan (or any plan for that matter) things don't always go smoothly — as recognized in recent shutdowns due to a global pandemic. Many of us lost interest in or access to gyms, rec centers, studios, and countless other locations that were integral to our plan. The loss of these facilities certainly created an obstacle for those who frequent and depend upon them. Drive and dedication are part of a strong mind, and they force us to come up with solutions, like doing your own research, working out at home, or using an app, virtual coach, or instructor.

Obstacles are not all equal (thank goodness). Some are the simple kinds: distraction, scheduling conflicts, sleepiness, etc. Once habit kicks in, these hiccups are typically less of a bother. Until then, however, our mental fortitude keeps us performing the actions on our wellness plan. A strong mind knows that continued action — water intake, food choices, exercise, and rest — is necessary to achieve the goals we've set for ourselves. So, resilience supports our wellness by keeping us on track, doing the work, and making the right choices (more often than not) no matter what size the obstacle may be!

You know that mental strength is important to your overall wellness, now how do you support your existing strength and continue to build it? First let's focus on supporting what you already have. Self-preservation plays a big role in this. This isn't a cop-out! Sometimes you just need to cut yourself a little slack. While this might sound like I'm negating what I said earlier, I'm not. It's a balancing act. You know the difference between a daydream that's distracting you from a workout and a solvable problem that's more important. Sleepiness is easier (and safer) to push through than real fatigue. Start by protecting your existing resilience then build some more!

The old use-it-or-lose-it adage pertains to all your faculties! While repetitious strength training builds your muscles, repetitious mental stimulation strengthens your mind! We accomplish this everyday through conversation, activity planning, creative endeavours, and problem-solving. These tasks vary in difficulty and all become easier with practice. Parents — remember the different stress levels you felt between your first and second child? I certainly do! For that matter, all stresses have fazed me less and less as I've matured (sounds nicer than *aged* — I'm cheesy, not cheese).

There are also many activities, games, and tools available to stimulate your mental muscle — your brain is an organ but *mental muscle* sounds more fun … there's my creative side.

My Grampa enjoyed mechanical puzzles, such as jigsaw and disentanglement puzzles — I still remember my excitement and pride having solved my first one, over thirty years ago. Rubik's Cube, nail puzzles, word searches, crosswords, sudoku, trivia, cryptic, math, and logic puzzles … there are so many to choose from. Just do a simple internet search!

Reading and writing is one of my favourite stimulation outlets — can you tell? Books come in so many styles and subjects — keeping Amazon, Indigo, and others in business. Not only is reading (and writing) stimulating for your mind, it also allows a creative outlet to assist you in self-preservation. While on the subject of creative endeavours, let's recognize some of those stimulating activities: drawing, painting, sculpting, model assembly, sewing, and more. Perhaps the physical activity of playing music and/or dancing is your thing. Sometimes creativity is simply rearranging a room.

Learning a new skill (like home renos during the pandemic) stimulates your brain. Earlier I referred to how much better I was able to deal with my second child after gaining Mom skills with my first. I'm sure that you'd agree, parenting is a skill! What new skills have you considered?

Games played independently or with others are fun ways to stimulate your brain. Solitaire, crazy eights, or gin rummy are classic card games. What about the seemingly endless varieties of board games, like checkers, chess, Trivial Pursuit, and Monopoly; or adult-type games, like Cards Against Humanity or What Do You Meme? Although I didn't always enjoy games growing up, they certainly have come a long way and I enjoy 'em now!

The above activities and many more, like conversation — one of my favourite pastimes — help to stimulate our minds, protecting and developing our mental strength. The stronger your mental muscle is, the better you're able to overcome obstacles with less worry or stress — keeping you in better spirits, ya know? Getting over these obstacles also keeps you progressing through the steps of your wellness plan even through adversity — body, mind, and spirit working together!

Agreed?

CHAPTER 7

You can change the way you think

In Part I we focused on changing your physical habits. I asked you to write down some wants and to start thinking about how you might achieve your goals. So guess where all change begins? In your mind, of course, which means a better understanding of how your mind works is paramount to changing the way you think so that you can make a real change in your life. In this chapter, we'll talk about how to change the way you *think* to change the way you *live*. Now that you know what your goals are (from chapter 1), it's time to think about what's stopping you from achieving them (limiting beliefs) and how you can change the way you think to get where you want to be (brainstorming an action plan).

From the time we're children, the way we think, the way we're *programmed*, is affected by our environment, parents, families, friends, peers, colleagues, communities, and experiences, but only *we* have control over *our minds*.

That means you can change the way you learn to think — the way your mind works. So those beliefs agreed to in your youth and throughout your life can change, if you decide to make that happen.

Perhaps some of your current beliefs aren't serving you well or are limiting you in some capacity. Consider what limiting beliefs are holding you back from your goals and write them in the space provided. For example, *It's too late in my life to start exercising. I don't have the time to exercise. I don't know what foods to eat.*

_____

_____

_____

_____

_____

_____

_____

_____

_____

_____

_____

_____

_____

_____

_____

_____

_____

By agreeing to these limiting beliefs you give them power. Fortunately, you can take that power back by changing your beliefs. Often it's as simple as turning a negative into a positive. For example, *It's too late in my life to start exercising* becomes *I'm so worthy of the strong and energized feeling that I gain from exercise.* Just imagine the accomplished feelings that accompany the action inspired by that statement. Try this yourself. Review your limiting beliefs and rewrite them in a positive way.

_____

_____

_____

_____

_____

_____

_____

_____

_____

_____

_____

_____

_____

_____

_____

_____

_____

Use these affirmations daily to remind yourself of your value. Post-it notes placed in plain sight, artwork, calendar events, or notes on your phone are great ways to surround yourself with positivity!

You can be more authentic in your actions and communication when you understand what's important to you. If you look at a list of values, some of them seem to jump off the page or evoke a strong feeling. Have a look at the following list and see what evokes a feeling in you. Circle or highlight those that do.

Acceptance	*Control*	*Focus*
Accuracy	*Cooperation*	*Foresight*
Adaptability	*Courtesy*	*Friendship*
Ambition	*Creativity*	*Fun*
Authenticity	*Dependability*	*Generosity*
Awareness	*Determination*	*Grace*
Balance	*Devotion*	*Gratitude*
Beauty	*Dignity*	*Growth*
Boldness	*Discipline*	*Health*
Bravery	*Eccentricity*	*Honesty*
Candour	*Effectiveness*	*Hope*
Certainty	*Empathy*	*Imagination*
Charity	*Endurance*	*Individuality*
Cleanliness	*Enthusiasm*	*Insight*
Commitment	*Equality*	*Inspiration*
Community	*Excellence*	*Integrity*
Compassion	*Experience*	*Intelligence*
Competence	*Family*	*Intensity*

Joy	*Presence*	*Spontaneity*
Justice	*Recognition*	*Stability*
Kindness	*Recreation*	*Strength*
Knowledge	*Respect*	*Success*
Leadership	*Responsibility*	*Sustainability*
Logic	*Reverence*	*Thought*
Love	*Rigour*	*Tolerance*
Loyalty	*Satisfaction*	*Toughness*
Maturity	*Security*	*Tradition*
Moderation	*Self-Reliance*	*Trust*
Motivation	*Sensitivity*	*Unity*
Optimism	*Service*	*Vigour*
Organization	*Significance*	*Wealth*
Originality	*Simplicity*	*Winning*
Patience	*Sincerity*	*Wisdom*
Peace	*Skill*	*Wit*
Persistence	*Solitude*	*Wonder*
Potential	*Spirit*	*Zip*

Some will likely be more powerful than others. Those ones are our core values and they can vary in priority or importance depending on the circumstance. For example, I value compassion and dependability, so if someone I care about cancels plans with me it could evoke a compassionate response or disappointment depending on our communication, the consistency of that behaviour, and how I'm feeling at the time. These values naturally develop or diminish as we age as a result of our life experiences. Also, you can choose to develop or diminish your values or beliefs through a committed decision and consistent, repetitious action. The task is simple yet not necessarily easy.

Changing the way you think requires strong stimuli, such as 1) a powerful life experience or 2) a committed and believed decision that is backed by action. Let's look at each of these:

A powerful life experience. The final wisdom that my mom left me with was to *own my emotions.* We were chatting in her room at Stedman Hospice (a beautiful and comfortable place to endure losing a loved one) when I asked her, "How are you feeling?" Her answer was, "I'm fabulous." You can imagine my disbelief since she was terminally ill with lung cancer, so I questioned her. She said, with a soft and gentle voice, "Just decide." It wasn't the first time I'd heard her use this phrase, since her consistent intention was to help me come to terms with any challenge that life brought. On this occasion, her intention was to help me come to terms with her death, which occurred two days later. You see, while you can't always control what happens around you, you do have absolute power over how you choose to feel about any given situation. Obviously the poignancy of this moment profoundly affected me, and I'm eternally grateful to her for teaching me this through example and simple explanation.

A committed and believed decision that is backed by action. Strong emotions often accompany powerful life experiences, and these serve as the energy required to change. Making an emotionalized decision has far greater power and potential than simply stating, "I want to be fit." What this means is that you've got to get happy, excited, grateful, etc. for what you want to achieve. You must state it as though it's already happened and *believe* it! Without your belief, it won't happen. How can you possibly take the action necessary to achieve a goal if some part of you doesn't believe it can or will happen? This is the power that your mind has over your actions. Furthermore, you've gotta write it down in a journal, in notes on your phone, or right here. For example, *I'm so excited to have two inches off my waistline. I can move more now that the bloated feeling is gone!* Writing this down can help keep your mind in a positive place and wanting more change because it feels so good!

_____

_____

_____

_____

_____

_____

_____

_____

_____

_____

_____

_____

_____

_____

_____

_____

_____

_____

_____

_____

_____

_____

_____

_____

_____

Saying it aloud and repeating it daily (at least) while believing what you're stating is paramount. What you actively think (what you *choose* to think) becomes — through repetition — your belief. If you want to change your body and you're repeating, *affirming*, that then you're more likely to make a choice that moves you toward your goal. If you've decided that you want a smaller waistline then you'll say no to those chips or that chocolate bar or whatever doesn't support your goal of a smaller waistline.

Upon development of your believed, exciting, or passionate decision about your primary want, you must then create a detailed action plan. Imagine taking a trip without GPS, Google maps, or an old-fashioned map.

Might be fun but you probably wouldn't end up where you intended. The same holds true for your personal wellness goals.

Brainstorming time! Write down actions that are necessary to achieve your goal. Don't be skimpy, write lots! For example, *I will exercise for 30 minutes daily. I will enjoy at least 3L of water daily.*

Ultimately, making improvements or changes in your life is not only possible but probable — you just have to make the commitment to change. Now let's take some time to really think about how to achieve those goals. On the following pages, try this exercise:

1. Write out an expansive list of wants without allowing yourself to feel limited in any way. (Remember, search your mind and don't hold back.)

2. Choose the most powerful one that elicits the greatest emotions (the one that gives you the *feels)* and devise a specific and detailed goal statement incorporating emotion and belief.

3. Establish an action plan by brainstorming all potential steps that will move you toward your goal and start it immediately!

4. Use your action plan to develop powerful and positive affirmations to support the establishment of new beliefs, actions, and therefore habits. Consistently replace all negative thoughts with positive ones.

5. Monitor progression toward the goal and make
    any necessary adjustments to your plan when
    required.

If you find this overwhelming, it can help to seek out
support, guidance, and accountability from trusted and
positive individuals or sources. But the first part of this
process is absolutely up to you, *Just Decide!*

_____

_____

_____

_____

_____

_____

_____

_____

_____

_____

_____

_____

_____

_____

_____

_____

_____

_____

_____

_____

_____

_____

_____

_____

_____

_____

_____

_____

_____

_____

_____

_____

_____

_____

_____

_____

_____

_____

_____

_____

_____

_____

_____

_____

_____

_____

_____

_____

_____

_____

_____

_____

_____

_____

_____

_____

_____

_____

_____

_____

_____

_____

_____

_____

_____

_____

_____

_____

_____

_____

_____

_____

_____

Here's where the big action comes in ... do what you planned! What good are directions in the bottom of a drawer? I'm a big fan of notes on my phone and just recently learned there's a ✅ option. It's fabulous for daily checklists! It's also easily edited so you can add or remove things as needed. While you can keep multiple checklists, it's important to remain focused on primary objectives in each aspect of your life. And the beauty of the checklist is that it's *repeatable*. Remember, repetition is necessary to create new and healthy habits. Use the list until it's no longer necessary for the creation of a particular habit. How will you know? You'll simply perform that task automatically, or "habitually." When that occurs, consider another necessary habit to develop and begin again!

---

1. Decide what to do.
2. Take immediate action!
3. Overcome obstacles (replace limiting beliefs with positive affirmations).
4. Assess and correct (repetition, trial and error).

Trial and error is a valuable way to get things done. If at first it doesn't work, simply change the plan!

Agreed?

A big part of successfully making change has to do with *attitude*. Your attitude is the way you choose to think, feel and behave about a situation or person, so it affects everything you do. Your attitude can change from second to second and year to year if you allow or encourage it. With persistent practice you can select what thoughts to honour and give space to in your mind. These active thoughts are what dictate and develop your feelings or beliefs, and those beliefs inspire your action. It became so clear to me when a mentor introduced me to the work of Bob Proctor. He speaks of our attitudes being organized into three interactive components: our thoughts, feelings, and actions (Gallagher 2016). I've reordered and interpreted this as follows: our body, mind, and spirit.

To adjust our attitudes, we need repetitive reminders from internal or external sources. Self-suggestion, self-control, and personal discipline are internally sourced and powerful but quite often not enough. External forces, like media, coworkers, our family, and friends (when chosen correctly) can offer positive reminders and redirection when our attitude is off course. That's important because we feel better when our thoughts and feelings support our actions. This is when our best work and development happens!

So how can you nurture and develop the attitude that best serves you? You've heard the saying "You can't pour from an empty cup." It's a favourite of mine. If you want to live with your ideal attitude then you ought to nurture and care for it. Find positivity and inspiration whenever and wherever possible. You know what *fills your cup*. Seek it out and fill 'er up!

Another key point is the avoidance, whenever possible, of negativity. To put it bluntly, don't take unnecessary shit! There are some rules and regulations that we conform to in our individual environments and in society as a whole. You get to decide which are necessary and which aren't. While externally imposed negativity can weigh you down, it doesn't have to. This goes back to the thoughts you choose to honour and allow to live in your mind. When someone is complaining to you, it isn't necessarily about you. It can often be a reflection of their past or current experiences, their thoughts and/or feelings. Internalizing that or taking it personally doesn't help anyone and simply leads to a feeling of unease. Not a good way to feel at all. Happily, there are tricks and tactics to avoid that feeling. One of them is *effective communication*.

Agreed?

CHAPTER 8
Effective communication

The previous chapter related to *internal* communication, aka self-suggestion. This is primary in the development of new beliefs and habits followed by consistent action to cement these habits. Also necessary for any new endeavour is *interactive* communication — quite simply, we don't live in isolation, and mutually beneficial relationships can propel us when we get stuck. Sharing our lives with others offers enrichment and a wide range of emotion that really makes it all worthwhile. So naturally, we find inspiration in those important to us. In other words, your external support system can help you make important wellness changes.

How you choose to communicate your goals will affect the level of support you receive from others. It isn't necessary to explain or justify your decisions to anyone, but if you choose to do so, why not ensure that your communication is as effective as possible?

Your words have great power to influence feelings, responses, and actions within yourself and others. If you've read *The Four Agreements* by Don Miguel Ruiz then you know that the first agreement is to "be impeccable with your word" (1997, 25) to yourself first then to others. So think it out for a bit, organize your thoughts, and decide what you'd like to share — be impeccable with your word.

Ultimately, when communicating, we must consider the following carefully:

1. **What we mean to say.** Our thoughts are often difficult to describe and to put into the right words. We have so much going on in our minds, sometimes it's hard to express ourselves, and what we want to say gets lost.

2. **What we actually say.** We all have different abilities when it comes to expressing our thoughts and feelings. As a result of this mind-to-mouth gap, sometimes we use the wrong words, and this leads to giving the wrong information or impression.

3. **What our audience hears.** What someone hears depends on so many things: what's going on in the room, whether the person is paying attention, how they're feeling at the time, and what might be distracting them. We have one mouth and two ears, so they ought to be used in the appropriate proportion — if you know me, I honestly do try.

4. **How our audience interprets what they hear.** Again, distractions, both internal and external,

can change the way people interpret your words. If, for example, some words were missed or misunderstood, that changes the message received. Or if someone is in a bad mood, they might assume a negative take on what you're saying. Personal feelings can really impact individual understanding.

All of these examples relate to face-to-face communication. When we text, email, or write, we remove tone, volume, pace, facial expression, body language, and so much more. The beauty of written communication is the potential time that goes into it and the ability to edit. Of course, this doesn't make it foolproof, because I'm currently writing from my feelings and experiences while you're reading from yours. It is certainly my intent to inspire, motivate, and empower you, but I have no control over how you will interpret this.

When we add false behaviour or absence of honesty and integrity (attitude misalignment) then our communication is nothing short of messed up. Our connections to each other are far deeper than verbal. Oftentimes (certainly for me) our facial expressions give us away. I'm one of those people who emote my feelings and thoughts through expression. While I have the ability to edit my words (usually), I'm not as successful as I would like to be at editing my expression. In this respect I'm certainly responding authentically, which is great, but I'm also intent on protecting others from an avoidably harsh response. I want to communicate with compassion as well as integrity. Being authentic doesn't necessitate being a bitch!

Communication is essential for the development of beliefs and habits. When we share our ideas by talking or writing, we're communicating. We can inspire and strengthen each other through thoughtful communication. Additionally, our family, friends, peers, and coaches (our external support system) help to keep us on track with our wellness goals. The other HUGE value of communication is the connection it supports and nurtures to loved ones and others. Being social creatures — each to varying degrees — offers far greater fulfillment than living a life of isolation.

Agreed?

PART III
Spirit

CHAPTER 9
What gives you the feels?

According to Google Dictionary, the definition of *spirit* is "the non-physical part of a person which is the seat of emotions and character; the soul." Sounds good to me! I loosely refer to my spirit as the part of me that has *the feels*. Consider the saying "If the spirit moves you." Of course this is a topic that elicits many feelings as a result of our passions. Our spirit, after all, is recognized and defined by many in a non-physical way. When a person seeks to understand the human spirit (not all do) they may come across words like *intellect, creativity, drive, passion, compassion*, and many others that are part of our core values. Think back to those that you highlighted earlier.

The understanding of your core values and being your authentic self helps you to better know yourself, make appropriate decisions, and take appropriate action. Your greatest personal development occurs when your *body* (action), *mind* (conscious and subconscious thoughts), and *spirit* (feelings and values) are working congruently with one another. Think about how you feel when you say or do something that isn't in keeping with your beliefs. How would you describe those feelings?

_____

_____

_____

_____

_____

_____

_____

_____

_____

_____

_____

_____

_____

_____

_____

_____

_____

_____

_____

_____

Now for the great *feels*. Consider times when you were thinking, feeling, and acting in alignment. This is also known as living an integral life, or *your actions matching your words*. We know that our thoughts direct our words and therefore our actions, so living a life of integrity is where the great *feels* come from. Choose a memory where this was clear to you. It doesn't have to be a game changer or monumental moment, just whatever comes to you. So pick one, close your eyes, and focus on it. Actually visualize it now.

So how does that feel? I imagine it makes you feel great! Write down those feelings.

_____

_____

_____

_____

_____

_____

_____

_____

_____

_____

_____

_____

_____

_____

_____

_____

_____

_____

_____

_____

_____

_____

_____

_____

_____

_____

_____

_____

_____

This is an example of living authentically or being your authentic self. To truly know and respect yourself above all others is paramount. This doesn't mean be selfish but rather focus on self-preservation and self-respect. I know that while I'm not alone in this belief, it's not universally shared ... I'm ok with that. I do *me*, and you do *you*.

When you work toward (and beyond) your personal development goals, you use your body, mind, and spirit. And throughout this process, you have to keep evaluating your success and make changes if something isn't working. *If at first you don't succeed, try, try again.* Often, this means overcoming negative feelings you may encounter along the way. Remember, use trial and error and actively practise new actions as best you can for 21 days.

1. Decide what to do.
2. Take immediate action!
3. Overcome obstacles (replace limiting beliefs with positive affirmations).
4. Assess and correct (repetition, trial and error).

Do you need to change your plan?

_____
_____
_____
_____
_____
_____
_____
_____
_____
_____
_____
_____
_____
_____
_____
_____
_____

Your body is responsible for your actions. Your mind is where ideas are created or planted, decided upon, believed in, and developed. Your spirit, the seat of emotions, is the fuel that drives your beliefs and actions. It's a real chicken-or-egg-first kinda question. Does your body act on things that your mind doesn't tell it to? When these things become habits, then yes it does. Of course they become habits because you decided in your mind to establish them and fueled the belief and action with powerful and positive emotions. It's just so reciprocal and effective how your body, mind, and spirit work together like a miraculous machine.

Agreed?

CHAPTER 10
Spiritual wellness

What is spirit? It's the part that gives you the *feels*, your internal light or energy, that which compels you to move. When a moment takes my breath, evokes a smile or laughter, then I feel it has touched my spirit in a positive or uplifting way. When I slump my shoulders or feel deflated then I'm experiencing a blow to my spirit. When you can't control things around you, your spirit is vulnerable, especially if you lack strength or wellness. Consider your feelings during the prolonged experience of the Covid-19 pandemic. Most of us have had feelings all over the emotional map.

Spiritual wellness is the preservation or protection of your spirit as well as knowing how to lift it up! Doing so gives your life greater fulfillment and better enables you to overcome obstacles. As mental strength is built through stimulation, so is spiritual wellness!

So how do you protect and preserve your spiritual wellness? This is where self-preservation plays a HUGE role.

The way you interact with people, your generosity and kindness, lifts your spirits. Remember my favourite saying? "You can't pour from an empty cup" — or as my son recently said to me, "I know, Mom, you have no fucks to give." Powerful and somewhat harsh, I know, but sometimes you've just gotta draw the line and restore your spirit to its fuller capacity before offering that precious commodity to others — even your children. Of course, this isn't new information, and you already know what fills your cup, but perhaps you'd like to do that more and could use a reminder of how valuable you are and how much you deserve it!

Those actions and things that give you the feels are what you need more of to continually stimulate and lift your spirit. Like *thinking* is stimulation for your mind, positive feelings are stimulation for your spirit. Even the little things, like time with family or friends, a tidy home (I know I'm not alone in this one), or a hug offer positive fuel to lift your spirit. I won't list all of mine because this is about you. The important thing is to recognize all the things that give you the feels and remember how super-duper important they are. A great writing exercise is to create a list of those things that fill your cup to remind you how many there are. (This is a wonderful resource for the times when you need it!) And I bet you'll get the feels simply by writing it.

_____

_____

_____

_____

I hope that exercise helped fuel your spirit and surprised you with great reminders! The things on your list are an important part of your day-to-day life, but the real substance comes from what you build your life around. Living a purposeful life is dependent upon knowing and being your authentic self — remember our core values from Part II? Look back on what you circled from the list and place an asterisk next to all that refer to positivity, generosity, gratitude — in general the happy ones. Did you mark most or all of them? Values like these are the spirit lifters, and when you honour them in making decisions about goals of all sizes — including your life's purpose — you're being your authentic self. Living a purposeful life is how you carry yourself through day-to-day activities, including the pursuit of your ultimate goal — that one thing!

Having a clear understanding of your ultimate purpose requires some self-reflection and sometimes counselling. Perhaps you've already considered your chief aim. Although I've always had some general idea that I enjoy helping others, I wasn't aware of my ultimate purpose until I was invited to really think about it. As you may remember from the introduction, my intention is to motivate and empower others to achieve what they desire. I apply this to everyone — my family, friends, and others seeking my direction, whether they are a regular part of my life or a flash in the pan.

You can live a purposeful life by making decisions and taking immediate action — no matter how small — overcoming obstacles, staying focused, and lifting your spirit while practising self-preservation. It might sound like a lot, but it offers a great amount of peace and fulfillment — beautiful things to strive for!

Agreed?

CHAPTER 11
We are all connected

Spirit isn't limited to us as individuals. We're surrounded by energy. It moves to us and through us. Google dictionary defines *ethos* as "the characteristic spirit of a culture, era, or community as manifested in its beliefs and aspirations." My interpretation: It's the spiritual atmosphere. Perhaps you have another interpretation?

So how is energy shared between living things and how can you use it? Let's talk a bit about the universal laws that are thought to be naturally and intuitively known, dating back through ancient cultures. They offer some explanation of the world we live in and how energy exists in it, and they guide or govern us — should we allow them to. The number of laws depends on the source you favour. I enjoy an interpretation offered by The Proctor Gallagher Institute, which I've summarized with some personal clarification (Gallagher 2019):

THE LAW OF ATTRACTION OR VIBRATION

This states that energy is always moving, or vibrating, and it's drawn to itself. More specifically, positive energy is drawn to the positive, and negative energy is drawn to the negative. Feelings *are* energy (remember they're our fuel). So positive feelings create and attract positive vibrations. Alternately, negative feelings create and attract negative vibrations. Like other strategies we've reviewed, we can edit — repeatedly if necessary — the energy we choose to draw to us. It begins with a decision! Consider an occasion when things seemed to go wrong … did focusing on that help to resolve the shit show or did it require a change of mind or attitude? Record a time when you turned negative feelings to positive.

_____

_____

_____

_____

_____

_____

_____

_____

_____

_____

_____

_____

_____

THE LAW OF PERPETUAL TRANSMUTATION

Thoughts are energy in its non-physical form, and when these thoughts are nourished by emotion, the body takes action. When we do this, we receive feedback from our senses — we experience sight, smell, taste, touch, and sound. We use this information and continue working until our idea manifests into its physical counterpart. Consider how fired up we can be by a great idea we have and the persistent action we take as a result!

THE LAW OF RHYTHM

You probably remember from school that every action has a reaction; to and fro, backward and forward, in and out. We see it in the rising and setting of the sun and moon, the ebb and flow of the tides, and the coming and going of the seasons. In us, it's the rhythmic swing of consciousness and unconsciousness. In the same way, low feelings allow us to recognize and appreciate high feelings. While we cannot perpetually have feelings of positivity, we can choose to think high in order to invite them back!

THE LAW OF RELATIVITY

We live in a big world, yet everything is connected. All things are relative to each other. A small tree is only small relative to a bigger tree. A sun*set* differs from and is relative to a sun*rise*. Everything is what it is. *We* make it big or small, dark or light, good or bad by comparing it to something else. When we compare ourselves to others, we're performing a disservice. Characteristics are personal. *Identical* and *individual* are beautifully opposing characteristics. We have unique strengths and challenges and would be better served developing what we choose to develop without comparing ourselves to others.

THE LAW OF POLARITY

And of course, everything has an opposite. Hot and cold, good and bad, inside and outside. If your belly button is three feet from the floor then the floor is also three feet from your belly button. Everything in your life is what it is and your perception makes it negative or positive by choice. Because it's your choices and not your circumstances that direct your life, would you not be better served by choosing positive thoughts?

THE LAW OF CAUSE AND EFFECT

Did you know that whatever you send to the universe comes back? Every cause has an effect and every effect was predicated by a cause. This action and reaction is perpetual and never-ending. Our power as individuals lies in our action. We must concentrate on cause, and the effect will take care of itself. Our control remains with us, not beyond. Take care of your body so that it may serve you well. Develop your mind so you can accomplish what you want. Respect your spirit so you can enjoy fulfillment.

THE LAW OF GENDER OR GESTATION

In the creative process, ideas have a gestation period before they are manifested into their physical counterpart.

A period of time must elapse while the ideas, or seeds, are nourished by the energy of emotionalized concentration. The length of this gestation period is directly affected by the level of concentration we apply. The implication here is that *you* have influence over the period between the sowing and reaping of your ideas.

What stood out from this discussion of energy and our world? Is there anything you might change about yourself to serve yourself and others better? Jot down your thoughts and feelings here.

_____

_____

_____

_____

_____

_____

_____

_____

_____

_____

_____

_____

_____

_____

_____

_____

_____

_____

The subject of a higher spirit is a very personal and often passionate topic. I imagine no two people completely agree about the meaning or definition of a higher spirit. I know I've yet to come across one explanation covering *spirit* that I'm in complete agreement with. And that's totally okay with me because I don't want all the answers at this time. What I do enjoy is a positive, respectful, and *spirited* conversation.

Our body, mind, and spirit are the sum of us as individuals, yet we live in a connected environment. Our connection — to each other, to nature, and to the universe — is the ultimate beauty that we call life, and nurturing and developing this connection serves to improve us as individuals and as a whole.

You can see your body, mind, and spirit agreements in the notes you made in this book. You may find them in a core value you listed or in a goal statement, an affirmation, or maybe a portion of a natural law. Return to the beginning and review the sections where notes were made. Is there repetition? That might indicate something is important to you. What statements or affirmations stand out? Understand that we're always evolving and agreements can change. Remember that agreements become natural or habitual through repetition, and these new agreements are the ultimate purpose of this book. Consider your current wants and record your agreements in the space provided on the next few pages. You may choose to categorize them into body, mind, and spirit, or not.

They're your agreements, so do as you will. You have lots of space, so creatively note your ideas and then edit them into clearly worded agreements. This will make the practice of agreements easier!

Agreed?

Yours in good health,

Carrie Brooks

_____

_____

_____

_____

_____

_____

_____

_____

_____

_____

_____

_____

_____

_____

_____

_____

_____

_____

_____

_____

_____

_____

_____

_____

_____

_____

_____

_____

_____

_____

_____

_____

_____

_____

_____

_____

_____

_____

_____

_____

_____

_____

_____

_____

_____

_____

_____

_____

_____

_____

_____

Acknowledgements

My aim upon waking each morning is to reflect on what I'm grateful for. It's not necessarily anything monumental, and some days are easier than others. For example, the first thing I think about is usually the comfort of my bed, then the sunrise, the love of my family … and my progress toward or achieving a goal. Allowing and nurturing positive thoughts or feelings just sets us up for happiness and success! What springs to your mind when contemplating gratitude?

As I'm sure you've recognized through what I've shared thus far, I like the people I spend my days with. I like what I do for a living. Over the years there have been a number of experiences that beautifully illustrated this, and I'd like to share some of them with you (with the names changed, of course).

When I met and began my time with Laurie, she was struggling to find happiness — so much, that the nickname "Dark Cloud" kinda stuck to her (I used it myself, until I shared it with Laurie). It should be mentioned that this nickname was actually picked out of a story she had shared with me. Laurie was a busy professional balancing a demanding career and the needs of a husband and two teens. As I like to do, I often spoke of the power of positivity and the law of attraction, a subject not new to Laurie. The brightest moment we shared was the day the clouds lifted. Her return to practising mindful positivity began to work for her, and she arrived one day as a ray of sunshine (my new and improved nickname for her). I was thrilled to see that she had found her beautiful smile.

Jill has played a very special role in my life for some time now. She has, many times, been the voice of reason, often appreciated … but not every time. I can, occasionally, be disagreeable. We've chatted about many things, easy-peasy conversations, experiences from funny to sad to extremely challenging. She has a kind and no-nonsense-type wisdom about her that has helped me through many situations and decisions in my life. She offers it with diplomacy, consideration, and great intellect. I'm consistently grateful for our conversations, from silly to serious, and the giggles and comfort that they bring!

Simon is a bright and charming professional I've always respected and he carries himself with integrity and compassion. Early on in our time together he was more reserved and private but had fun pushing through a workout — he even smiled here and there. When he eventually began sharing (through shortness of breath in a fabulous Columbian accent), I felt I'd gotten over a bit of a hurdle and was flattered and grateful for his trust. Sometimes the tough nuts are the most rewarding to crack! After sharing my concerns about my daughter's upcoming scoliosis surgery some years ago (she's since successfully recuperated), it was his sympathetic and calming tone that brought me so much comfort, and I will always remember it fondly.

What a great character Pete is. The sparkle in his eyes and his wild (somewhat inappropriate) sense of humour never cease to amaze and amuse me. Not just a funny guy, he's also full of great advice. Our conversations almost always involve laughter, even while he's calling me a bully and sharing that sentiment with anyone who will listen. Over the years we've gotten closer, and I'm grateful to also call him a good friend who I know I can count on!

Ah Rachel ... she began as any other client, all special in their unique ways. Rachel wasn't a huge fan of the gym, but she put in the time and had great success with her transformation — all the while keeping me posted about what she enjoyed ... and what she didn't, lol. She tends to play things close to the vest, but feedback is important so she would update me on anything relevant. It would be putting it mildly to say I was surprised when Rachel announced (while dismounting the hack squat machine) that we should just be friends instead of this working-out shit. Seems she was right 'cause she's been like an octopus stuck to my face (an endearing euphemism we like) for roughly a decade now.

What a positive personality Cindy has … man oh man, do I ever look forward to our sessions. We clicked (her term) instantly. We're like-minded, and I'm quite sure she's taught me much more than I've taught her. I see Cindy as a limitless individual and I believe she sees others the same way. Our conversations flow so naturally and almost always focus on positivity and possibilities. My favourite moments are the ah-ha moments we seem to have regularly. Casually sharing thoughts that lead to simultaneous smiles and laughter … what joy!

Bambi is so honest and authentic. I have such respect and admiration for her. If she says it, she means it and if she means it, she says it. This doesn't mean that she's hurtful, quite the opposite is true. She has this amazing ability to share her thoughtful insights, when asked or inspired to do so, in a non-invasive way. Her smile and laughter are so real and infectious … her singing voice is pretty fab too! I'm grateful to have known her for years and intend to maintain our friendship for many more to come.

Penny is a kind and loving soul. She sees the good in others and celebrates it with enthusiasm. It would be challenging to find time with her unenjoyable … unless you're a devout grump (although she'd likely bring a grump around too). Her stories are nothing short of epic and powerful … she has brought tears to my eyes as a result of emotions, both happy and sad.

Maddy is quite simply the perfect picture of kindness. She truly has patience and kind words for everyone along with sparkling eyes and a beautiful smile. Always striving for self-improvement while caring for the needs of others is something that makes her an inspiration to me. Our conversations feel so connected and uplifting. We are so often in agreement about the beautiful power of a positive mind and the way it directs our actions and beliefs!

Such a kind, wise, and happy person is how I would best describe Kathy. I learned right off the hop what a shrewd and polite negotiator she was when she asked to amend the personal training contract — cancelling it should I ever leave the gym. Although I knew it wouldn't be accepted by management, it felt so complimentary nonetheless. In the years that have passed since then, her importance in my life has grown significantly and I'm grateful to call her a close friend as well as a client.

Henry was the client who first illustrated to me the benefit that I offered to all clients, including those who were highly educated such as he. While directing him (one of my first clients) through an exercise, I mentioned how it seemed odd that I was educating him, an established medical professional. Responding with sincerity and a kind tone (his normal communication style), he indicated that my caring direction was of great value to him as weight training was outside the scope of his years of education and training.

Abby is another inspirational person whose conversation I find stimulating. She is so confident, wise, and well-spoken that our time together seems to fly by.

We talk endlessly about physical well-being, personal development, and the importance of a positive attitude. One recent and humorous conversation left me somewhat stumped by her specific and slightly limiting exercise requests. I'm not good at editing my facial expressions, and Abby's sympathetic chuckle was amusing for us both. I think the reason that this stands out is that it's the first conversation we've had in roughly five years that had a bit of a lull in it.

Mindy is another one of those positive individuals who also turned into a good friend. I've watched her grow with class and poise, through both adversity and positive life experiences. I'm grateful to her for speaking passionately about positivity even before I was ready to believe it. Dream, Believe & Achieve is a general sentiment that was introduced to me by her over ten years ago, and I'm so happy to now better understand the power of a positive attitude.

For many years Jenny has made me laugh. While she didn't begin her health journey with whole-hearted conviction, she has certainly improved greatly. Our time together almost always includes laughter because Jenny can really spin a yarn! Watching her mature into a strong, caring, and beautiful wife and mom, who consistently makes time for self-improvement as well as her family and others, makes me feel proud of this dear friend.

Linda experienced a whole transformation. During our first sessions together when she was a teenager, she was disinterested, to put it mildly, and lasted only a few weeks. Upon her return to the gym two years later she had developed into a mature, positive, and dedicated young woman who was a pleasure to train. Her hard work and consistency yielded her a loss of almost 100 pounds and a gain of greater strength, mobility, and confidence that she continues to wear so well!

It's so easy to watch Amanda's enjoyment of working out. While she doesn't always begin our sessions that way, she's grinning with pride by the end. Consistently accommodating and up for whatever challenge I present, she's another shining example that perseverance builds personal strength, character, and a glowing feeling of accomplishment.

In our years together, Janine helped me to better understand compassion. It wasn't a proud moment for me when I wasn't "reading the room" or aware of her disposition one afternoon. When I chuckled as a result of her make-up application prior to our session, she calmly took my hand, and I knew instantly by her expression and tone that she needed that at the moment. Her endless kindness, strength, and compassion remain clear in my memory, and my hope is that she remembers me as fondly as I remember her.

With a quick wit and a cheerful smile, Annie has been a pleasure to coach the past few years. She moves through our workouts with a smile and a little sweat, and she's always got a story or two to share. As we're approaching the completion of our sessions, I know that

I'll miss our jovial conversations but I'll get to keep seeing her smile as she continues her exercises for years to come.

Martha enjoyed almost every exercise that I taught her and executed them well and with a smile. Her level of personal dedication was shown by her consistent attendance at our weekly sessions. Always wanting to be challenged, she allowed me the opportunity to flex my creative muscles. Thankfully, through the power of social media, I still enjoy "seeing" Martha and others who have moved away.

Little nuggets of wisdom and laughter have continued to educate me and build my character ... hence my gratitude for your attitude.

References

BOOKS

Fung, Dr Jason. 2016. *The Obesity Code: Unlocking the Secrets of Weight Loss*. Brunswick: Scribe.

Hill, Napolean. 1937. *Think and Grow Rich*. Meriden, CT: The Ralston Society.

Ruiz, Miguel. 1997. *The Four Agreements: A Practical Guide to Personal Freedom*. San Rafael, CA: Amber-Allen Publishing.

WEBSITES

Bjarnadottir, Adda. 2020. "How Drinking More Water Can Help You Lose Weight." Healthline. Healthline Media, December 14, 2020. https://www.healthline.com/nutrition/drinking-water-helps-with-weight-loss.

Gallagher, Sandy. 2016. "The Truth About Your Attitude." Proctor Gallagher Institute, February 22, 2016.

https://www.proctorgallagherinstitute.com/9355/the-truth-about-your-attitude.

Gallagher, Sandy. 2019. "Seven Universal Laws at a Glance." Proctor Gallagher Institute, May 6, 2019. https://www.proctorgallagherinstitute.com/35331/seven-universal-laws-at-a-glance.

Mangano, Meg. 2011. "What Happens to the Excess Food?" RejoovWellness, August 25, 2011. https://rejoovwellness.com/1143/.

Mawer, Rudy. 2019. "11 Ways to Boost Human Growth Hormone (HGH) Naturally." Healthline. Healthline Media, September 23, 2019. https://www.healthline.com/nutrition/11-ways-to-increase-hgh.

Silver, Natalie. 2020. "Why Is Water Important? 16 Reasons to Drink Up." Healthline. Healthline Media, July 1, 2020. https://www.healthline.com/health/food-nutrition/why-is-water-important.

Still, Jennifer. 2019. "Types of Water: 9 Different Sources and Brands, Plus Benefits & Risks." Healthline. Healthline Media, March 8, 2019. https://www.healthline.com/health/food-nutrition/nine-types-of-drinking-water.

Virgin, JJ. 2013. "Why Snacking Can Stall Fat Loss and Fast Metabolism." HuffPost. HuffPost, May 27, 2013. http://www.huffpost.com/entry/snacking-weight-loss_b_2940998.

CPSIA information can be obtained
at www.ICGtesting.com
Printed in the USA
LVHW091632090521
686930LV00004B/316

9 781771 804882